My Alkaline Snacks and Salads Cookbook

A collection of 50 Alkaline Dishes for your Healthy Break

Isaac Vinson

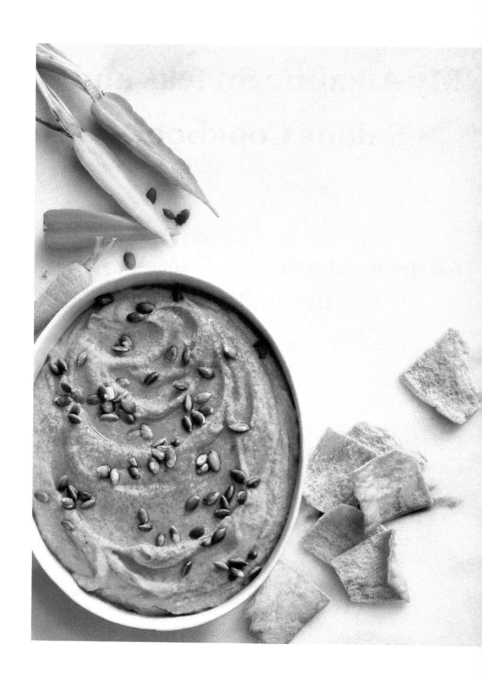

Table of Contents

Orange- Spiced Pumpkin Hummus

Preparation Time: 2 minutes
Cooking Time: 5 minutes
Servings: 4 cups

Ingredients :
- 1 tablespoon maple syrup

- 1/2 teaspoon salt

- 1 can (16oz.) garbanzo beans,

- 1/8 teaspoon ginger or nutmeg

- 1 cup canned pumpkin Blend,

- 1/8 teaspoon cinnamon

- 1/4 cup tahini

- 1 tablespoon fresh orange juice

- Pinch of orange zest, for garnish

- 1 tablespoon apple cider vinegar

Directions:

Mix all the Ingredients to a food processor blender and blend until slightly chunky.

Serve right away and enjoy!

Nutrition:

91 calories

2.9g fat

5g total carbohydrates

2g protein

Cinnamon Maple Sweet Potato Bites

Preparation Time: 5 minutes

Cooking Time: 25 minutes

Servings: 3 to 4

Ingredients :

• ½ teaspoon corn-starch

• 1 teaspoon cinnamon

• 4 medium sweet potatoes, then peeled, and cut into bite-si⬚ cubes

• 2 to 3 tablespoons maple syrup

• 3 tablespoons butter, melted

Directions:

1. Transfer the potato cubes to a Ziploc bag and add in ⬚ tablespoons of melted butter. Seal and shake well until t⬚ potato cubes are coated with butter.

2. Add in the remaining Ingredients and shake again.

3. Transfer the potato cubes to a parchment-lined baking she⬚ Cubes shouldn't be stacked on one another.

. Sprinkle with cinnamon, if needed, and bake in a preheated ven at 425°F for about 25 to 30 minutes, stirring once during ooking.

. Once done, take them out and stand at room temperature. njoy!

Nutrition:

36 calories

7.4g fat

1.8g total carbohydrates

.1g protein

Cheesy Kale Chips

Preparation Time: 3 minutes
Cooking Time: 12 minutes
Servings: 4

Ingredients :

• 3 tablespoons Nutritional yeast

• 1 head curly kale, washed, ribs

• 3/4 teaspoon garlic powder

• 1 tablespoon olive oil

• 1 teaspoon onion powder

• Salt, to taste

Directions:

1. Line cookie sheets with parchment paper.

2. Drain the kale leaves and spread on a paper removed an
leaves torn into chip-

3. towel. Then, kindly transfer the leaves to a bowl and size
pieces

add in 1 teaspoon onion powder, 3 tablespoons Nutritional ast, 1 tablespoon olive oil, and 3/4

teaspoon garlic powder. Mix with your hands.

Spread the kale onto prepared cookie sheets. They shouldn't uch each other.

Bake into a preheated oven for about 350 F for about 10to 12 inutes.

Once crisp, take out from the oven, and sprinkle with a bit of lt. Serve and enjoy!

utrition:

calories

; fat

; total carbohydrates

; protein

Lemon Roasted Bell Pepper

Preparation Time: 10 minutes
Cooking Time: 5 minutes
Servings: 4

Ingredients :

• 4 bell peppers

• 1 teaspoon olive oil

• 1 tablespoon mango juice

• 1/4 teaspoon garlic, minced

• 1 teaspoons oregano

• 1 pinch salt

• 1 pinch pepper

Directions:

1. Start heating the Air Fryer to 390 degrees F

2. Place some bell pepper in the Air fryer

3. Drizzle it with the olive oil and air fry for 5 minutes

4. Take a serving plate and transfer it

Take a small bowl and add garlic, oregano, mango juice, salt, d pepper

Mix them well and drizzle the mixture over the peppers

Serve and enjoy!

utrition:

lories: 59 kcal

rbohydrates: 6 g

t: 5 g

otein: 4 g

Subtle Roasted Mushrooms

Preparation Time: 10 minutes

Cooking Time: 5 minutes

Servings: 4

Ingredients :

• 2 teaspoons mixed Alkaline Friendly herbs

• 1 tablespoon olive oil

• 1/2 teaspoon garlic powder

• 2 pounds mushrooms

• 2 tablespoons date sugar

Directions:

1. Wash mushrooms and turn dry in a plate of mixed green spinner

2. Quarter them and put in a safe spot

3. Put garlic, oil, and spices in the dish of your oar type air fryer

4. Warmth for 2 minutes

5. Stir it.

. Add some mushrooms and cook 25 minutes

. Then include vermouth and cook for 5 minutes more

. Serve and enjoy!

Nutrition:

Calories: 94 kcal

Carbohydrates: 3 g

Fat: 8 g

Protein: 2 g.

Fancy Spelt Bread

Preparation Time: 10 minutes

Cooking Time: 5 minutes

Servings: 4

Ingredients :

• 1 cup spring water

• 1/2 cup of coconut milk

• 3 tablespoons avocado oil

• 1 teaspoon baking soda

• 1 tablespoon agave nectar

• 4 and 1/2 cups spelt flour

• 1 and 1/2 teaspoon salt

Directions:

1. Pre-heat your Air Fryer to 355 degrees F

2. Take a big bowl and add baking soda, salt, flour whisk well

3. Add 3/4 cup of water, plus coconut milk, oil and mix well

Sprinkle your working surface with flour, add dough to the our

Roll well

Knead for about three minutes, adding small amounts of flour until dough is a nice ball

Place parchment paper in your cooking basket

Lightly grease your pan and put the dough inside

Transfer into Air Fryer and bake for 30 minutes until done

). Remove then insert a stick to check for doneness

. If done already serve and enjoy, if not, let it cook for a few inutes more

utrition:

alories: 203 kcal

arbohydrates: 37 g

at: 4g

rotein: 7 g

Crispy Crunchy Hummus

Preparation Time: 10 minutes

Cooking Time: 10-15 minutes

Servings: 4

Ingredients :
- 1/2 a red onion

- 2 tablespoons fresh coriander

- 1/4 cup cherry tomatoes

- 1/2 a red bell pepper

- 1 tablespoon dulse flakes

- Juice of lime

- Salt to taste

- 3 tablespoons olive oil

- 2 tablespoons tahini

- 1 cup warm chickpeas

Directions:

1. Prepare your Air Fryer cooking basket

Add chickpeas to your cooking container and cook for 10-15 inutes, making a point to continue blending them every once a while until they are altogether warmed

Add warmed chickpeas to a bowl and include tahini, salt, lime

Utilize a fork to pound chickpeas and fixings in a glue until ıooth

Include hacked onion, cherry tomatoes, ringer pepper, dulse ops, and olive oil

Blend well until consolidated

Serve hummus with a couple of cuts of spelt bread

utrition:

lories: 95 kcal

rbohydrates: 5 g

t: 5 g

otein: 5 g

Chick Pea And Kale Dish

Preparation Time: 10 minutes
Cooking Time: 25-30 minutes

Servings: 4

Ingredients :

- 2 cups chickpea flour

- 1/2 cup green bell pepper, diced

- 1/2 cup onions, minced

- 1 tablespoon oregano

- 1 tablespoon salt

- 1 teaspoon cayenne

- 4 cups spring water

- 2 tablespoons Grape Seed Oil

Directions:

1. Boil spring water in a large pot

2. Lower heat into medium and whisk in chickpea flour

. Add some minced onions, diced green bell pepper, seasoning to the pot and cook for 10 minutes

. Cover dish using a baking sheet, grease with oil

. Pour batter into the sheet and spread with a spatula

. Cover with another sheet

. Transfer to a fridge and chill, for 20 minutes

. Remove from freezer and cut batter into fry shapes

. Preheat the Air Fryer, to 385 degrees F

0. Transfer fries into the cooking basket, lightly greased and cover with parchment

1. Bake for about 15 minutes, flip and bake for 10 minutes more until golden brown

2. Serve and enjoy!

Nutrition:

Calories: 271 kcal

Carbohydrates: 28 g

Fat: 15 g

Protein: 9 g

Zucchini Chips

Preparation Time: 10 minutes

Cooking Time: 12-15 minutes

Servings: 4

Ingredients :

• Salt as needed

• Grape seed oil as needed

• 6 zucchinis

Directions:

1. Into 330 F, pre heat the Air Fryer

2. Wash zucchini, slice zucchini into thin strips

3. Put slices in a bowl and add oil, salt, and toss

4. Spread over the cooking basket, fry for 12-15 minutes

5. Serve and enjoy!

Nutrition:

Calories: 92 kcal

Carbohydrates: 6 g

Fat: 7 g

Protein: 2 g

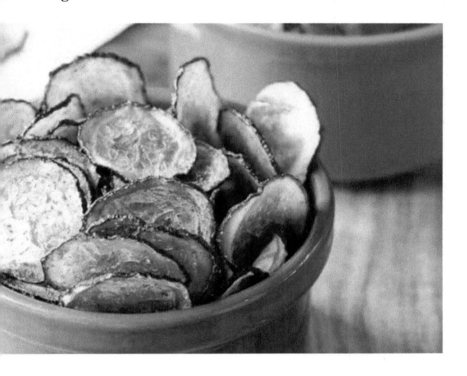

Classic Blueberry Spelt Muffins

Preparation Time: 10 minutes
Cooking Time: 12-15 minutes

Servings: 4

Ingredients :

- 1/4 sea salt

- 1/3 cup maple syrup

- 1 teaspoon baking powder

- 1/2 cup sea moss

- 3/4 cup spelt flour

- 3/4 cup Kamut flour

- 1 cup hemp milk

- 1 cup blueberries

Directions:

1. Into 380 degrees F pre heat Air Fryer

2. Take your muffin tins and gently grease them

Take a bowl and add flour, syrup, salt, baking powder, amless and mix well

Add milk and mix well

Fold in blueberries

Pour into muffin tins

Transfer to the cooking basket, bake for 20-25 minutes until cely baked

Serve and enjoy!

utrition:

lories: 217 kcal,

rbohydrates: 32 g

t: 9 g

otein: 4 g

Genuine Healthy Crackers

Preparation Time: 10 minutes

Cooking Time: 12-15 minutes

Servings: 4

Ingredients :

• 1/2 cup Rye flour

• 1 cup spelt flour

• 2 teaspoons sesame seed

• 1 teaspoon agave syrup

• 1 teaspoon salt

• 2 tablespoons grapeseed oil

• 3/4 cup spring water

Directions:

1. Into 330 degrees F, Preheat the Air Fryer

2. Take a medium bowl and add all Ingredients, mix well

3. Make dough ball

. Prepare a place for rolling out the dough, cover with a piece of parchment

. Lightly grease paper with grape seed oil, place dough

. Roll out, dough with a rolling pin, add more flour if needed

. Take a shape cutter and cut dough into squares

. Place squares in Air Fryer cooking basket

. Brush with more oil

0. Sprinkle salt

1. Bake for 10-15 minutes until golden

2. Let it cool, serve, and enjoy!

Nutrition:

alories: 226 kcal

arbohydrates: 41 g

at: 3 g

rotein: 11 g

Alkaline Tortilla Chips

Preparation Time: 10 minutes

Cooking Time: 8-12 minutes

Servings: 4

Ingredients :

• 2 cups of spelt flour

• 1 teaspoon of salt

• 1/2 cup of spring water

• 1/3 cup of grapeseed oil

Directions:

1. Preheat your Air Fryer into 320 degrees F

2. Take the food processor then add salt, flour, and process well for 15 seconds

3. Gradually add grapeseed oil until mixed

4. Keep mixing until you have a nice dough

5. Formulate work surface and cover in a piece of parchment, sprinkle flour

Knead the dough for 1-2 minutes

Grease cooking basket with oil

Transfer dough on the cooking basket, brush oil and sprinkle
lt

Cut dough into 8 triangles

. Bake for about 8-12 minutes until golden brown

. Serve and enjoy once done!

utrition:

lories: 288 kcal

rbohydrates: 18 g

it: 17 g

otein: 16 g

Pumpkin Spice Crackers

Preparation Time: 10 minutes
Cooking Time: 30 minutes
Servings: 06

Ingredients :

- 1⁄3 cup coconut flour

- 2 tablespoons pumpkin pie spice

- ¾ cup sunflower seeds

- ¾ cup flaxseed

- 1⁄3 cup sesame seeds

- 1 tablespoon ground psyllium husk powder

- 1 teaspoon sea salt

- 3 tablespoons coconut oil, melted

- 11⁄3 cups alkaline water

Directions:

1. Set your oven to 300 degrees F.

2. Combine all dry Ingredients in a bowl.

Add water and oil to the mixture and mix well.

Let the dough stay for 2 to 3 minutes.

Spread the dough evenly on a cookie sheet lined with rchment paper.

Bake for 30 minutes.

Reduce the oven heat to low and bake for another 30 minutes.

Crack the bread into bite-size pieces.

Serve

utrition:

lories 248

tal Fat 15.7 g

turated Fat 2.7 g

olesterol 75 mg

dium 94 mg

tal Carbs 0.4 g

ber 0g

gar 0 g

otein 24.9 g

Spicy Roasted Nuts

Preparation Time: 10 minutes

Cooking Time: 15 minutes

Servings: 4

Ingredients :

• 8 oz. pecans or almonds or walnuts

• 1 teaspoon sea salt

• 1 tablespoon olive oil or coconut oil

• 1 teaspoon ground cumin

• 1 teaspoon paprika powder or chili powder

Directions:

1. Add all the Ingredients to a skillet.

2. Roast the nuts until golden brown.

3. Serve and enjoy.

Nutrition:

Calories 287

Total Fat 29.5 g

Saturated Fat 3 g

Cholesterol 0 mg

Total Carbs 5.9 g

Sugar 1.4g

Fiber 4.3 g

Sodium 388 mg

Protein 4.2 g

Wheat Crackers

Preparation Time: 10 minutes
Cooking Time: 20 minutes
Servings: 4

Ingredients :

• 1 3/4 cups almond flour

• 1 1/2 cups coconut flour

• 3/4 teaspoon sea salt

• 1/3 cup vegetable oil

• 1 cup alkaline water

• Sea salt for sprinkling

Directions:

1. Set your oven to 350 degrees F.

2. Mix coconut flour, almond flour and salt in a bowl.

3. Stir in vegetable oil and water. Mix well until smooth.

4. Spread this dough on a floured surface into a thin sheet.

5. Cut small squares out of this sheet.

Arrange the dough squares on a baking sheet lined with parchment paper.

For about 20 minutes, bake until light golden in color.

Serve.

Nutrition:

Calories 64

Total Fat 9.2 g

Saturated Fat 2.4 g

Cholesterol 110 mg

Sodium 276 mg

Total Carbs 9.2 g

Fiber 0.9 g

Sugar 1.4 g

Protein 1.5 g

Potato Chips

Preparation Time: 10 minutes

Cooking Time: 20 minutes

Servings: 4

Ingredients :

• 1 tablespoon vegetable oil

• 1 potato, sliced paper thin

• Sea salt, to taste

Directions:

1. Toss potato with oil and sea salt.

2. Spread the slices in a baking dish in a single layer.

3. Cook in a microwave for 5 minutes until golden brown.

4. Serve.

Nutrition:

Calories 80

Total Fat 3.5 g

turated Fat 0.1 g

olesterol 320 mg

dium 350 mg

tal Carbs 11.6 g

er 0.7 g

gar 0.7 g

otein 1.2 g

Zucchini Pepper Chips

Preparation Time: 10 minutes
Cooking Time: 15 minutes
Servings: 04

Ingredients :

• 1 **Servings:** cups vegetable oil

• 1 teaspoon garlic powder

• 1 teaspoon onion powder

• 1/2 teaspoon black pepper

• 3 tablespoons crushed red pepper flakes

• 2 zucchinis, thinly sliced

Directions:

1. Mix oil with all the spices in a bowl.

2. Add zucchini slices and mix well.

3. Transfer the mixture to a Ziplock bag and seal it.

4. Refrigerate for 10 minutes.

5. Spread the zucchini slices on a greased baking sheet.

. Bake for 15 minutes

. Serve.

Nutrition:

Calories 172

Total Fat 11.1 g

Saturated Fat 5.8 g

Cholesterol 610 mg

Sodium 749 mg

Total Carbs 19.9 g

Fiber 0.2 g

Sugar 0.2 g

Protein 13.5 g

Kale Crisps

Preparation Time: 10 minutes

Cooking Time: 10 minutes

Servings: 04

Ingredients :

• 1 bunch kale, remove the stems, leaves torn into even pieces

• 1 tablespoon olive oil

• 1 teaspoon sea salt

Directions:

1. Set your oven to 350 degrees F. Layer a baking sheet with parchment paper.

2. Spread the kale leaves on a paper towel to absorb all the moisture.

3. Toss the leaves with sea salt, and olive oil.

4. Kindly spread them, on the baking sheet and bake for 10 minutes.

5. Serve.

Nutrition:

Calories 113

Total Fat 7.5 g

Saturated Fat 1.1 g

Cholesterol 20 mg

Sodium 97 mg

Total Carbs 1.4 g

Fiber 0 g

Sugar 0 g

Protein 1.1g

Carrot Chips

Preparation Time: 5 minutes

Cooking Time: 12 minutes

Servings: 4

Ingredients :

• 4 carrots, washed, peeled and sliced

• 2 teaspoons extra-virgin olive oil

• 1/4 teaspoon sea salt

Directions:

1. Set your oven to 350 degrees F.

2. Toss carrots with salt and olive oil.

3. Spread the slices into two baking sheets in a single layer.

4. Bake for 6 minutes on upper and lower rack of the oven.

5. Switch the baking racks and bake for another 6 minutes.

6. Serve.

Nutrition:

Calories 153

Total Fat 7.5 g

Saturated Fat 1.1 g

Cholesterol 20 mg

Sodium 97 mg

Total Carbs 20.4 g

Fiber 0 g

Sugar 0 g

Protein 3.1g

Pita Chips

Preparation Time: 5 minutes
Cooking Time: 12 minutes
Servings: 4

Ingredients :

• 12 pita bread pockets, sliced into triangles

• 1/2 cup olive oil

• 1/2 teaspoon ground black pepper

• 1 teaspoon garlic salt

• 1/2 teaspoon dried basil

• 1 teaspoon dried chervil

Directions:

1. Set your oven to 400 degrees F.

2. Toss pita with all the remaining Ingredients in a bowl.

3. Spread the seasoned triangles on a baking sheet.

4. Bake for 7 minutes until golden brown.

5. Serve with your favourite hummus.

Nutrition:

Calories 201

Total Fat 5.5 g

Saturated Fat 2.1 g

Cholesterol 10 mg

Sodium 597 mg

Total Carbs 2.4 g

Fiber 0 g

Sugar 0 g

Protein 3.1g

Sweet Potato Chips

Preparation Time: 5 minutes

Cooking Time: 5 minutes

Servings: 4

Ingredients :

• 1 sweet potato, thinly sliced

• 2 teaspoons olive oil, or as needed

• Coarse sea salt, to taste

Directions:

1. Toss sweet potato with oil and salt.

2. Spread the slices in a baking dish in a single layer.

3. Cook in a microwave for 5 minutes until golden brown.

4. Serve.

Nutrition:

Calories 213

Total Fat 8.5 g

turated Fat 3.1 g

nolesterol 120 mg

odium 497 mg

otal Carbs 22.4 g

ber 0 g

igar 0 g

rotein 0.1g

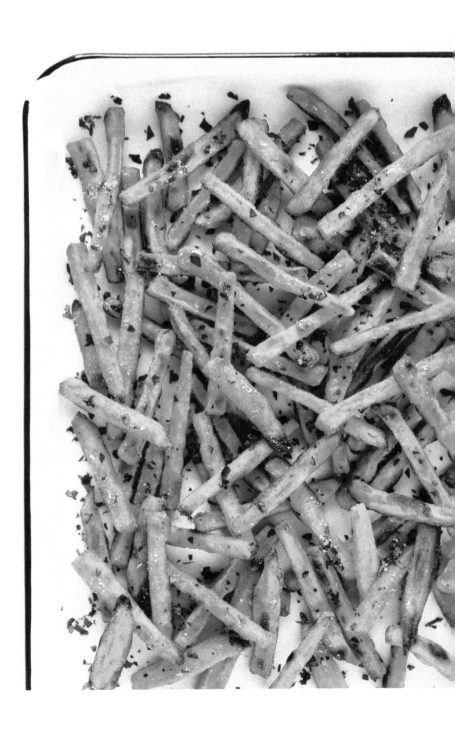

Kale Pesto's Pasta

Preparation Time: 10 minutes

Cooking Time: 0 minutes

Servings: 1-2

Ingredients :

bunch of kale

2 cups of fresh basil

1/4 cup of extra virgin olive oil

1/2 cup of walnuts

2 limes, freshly squeezed

Sea salt and chili pepper

1 zucchini, noodle (spiralizer)

Optional: garnish with chopped asparagus, spinach leaves, and tomato.

Directions:

The night before, soak the walnuts in order to improve absorption.

2. Put all the recipe Ingredients in a blender and blend until th
consistency of the cream is reached.

3. Add the zucchini noodles and enjoy.

Nutrition:

Calories: 55

Carbohydrates: 9 g

Fat: 1.2g

Cranberry And Brussels Sprouts With Dressing

Preparation Time: 10 minutes

Cooking Time: 0 minute

Servings: 4

Ingredients :

Ingredients for the dressing

⅓ cup extra-virgin olive oil

2 tbsp. apple cider vinegar

1 tbsp. pure maple syrup

Juice of 1 orange

½ tbsp. dried rosemary

1 tbsp. scallion, whites only

 Pinch sea salt

For the salad

• 1 bunch scallions, greens only, finely chopped

• 1 cup Brussels sprouts, stemmed, halved, and thinly sliced

• ½ cup fresh cranberries

• 4 cups fresh baby spinach

Directions:

1. To make the dressing: In a bowl, whisk the dressing Ingredients.

2. To make the salad: Add the scallions, Brussels sprouts, cranberries, and spinach to the bowl with the dressing.

3. Combine and serve.

Nutrition:

Calories: 267

Fat: 18g

Carbohydrates: 26g

Protein: 2g

Alkaline Vegetable Salad

Preparation Time: 10 minutes

Cooking Time: 0 minutes

Servings: 1-2

Ingredients :

4 cups each of raw spinach and romaine lettuce

2 cups each of cherry tomatoes, sliced cucumber, chopped baby carrots and chopped red, orange and yellow bell pepper

1 cup each of chopped broccoli, sliced yellow squash, zucchini and cauliflower.

Directions:

Wash all these vegetables.

Mix in a large mixing bowl and top off with a non-fat or low-fat dressing of your choice.

Nutrition:

Calories: 48

Carbohydrates: 11g

Protein: 3g

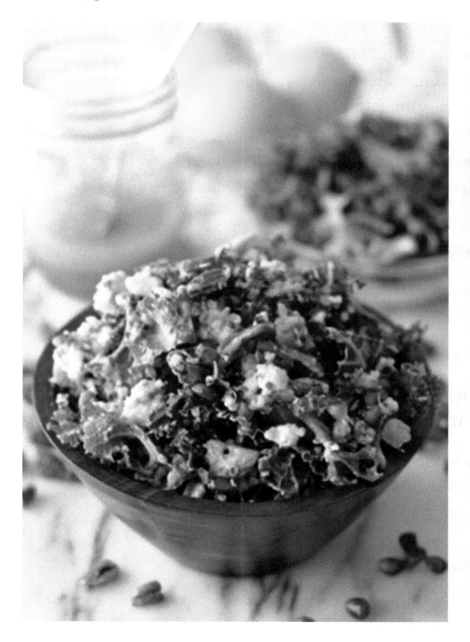

Alkaline Spring Salad

Preparation Time: 10 minutes

Cooking Time: 0 minutes

Servings: 1-2

Eating seasonal fruits and vegetables is a fabulous way of taking care of yourself and the environment at the same time. This alkaline-electric salad is delicious and nutritious.

Ingredients :

2 cups seasonal approved greens of your choice

1 cup cherry tomatoes

1/4 cup walnuts

1/4 cup approved herbs of your choice

For the dressing:

3-4 key limes

1 tbsp. of homemade raw sesame

Sea salt and cayenne pepper

Directions:

1. First, get the juice of the key limes. In a small bowl, whis together the key lime juice with the homemade raw sesam "tahini" butter. Add sea salt and cayenne pepper, to taste.

2. Cut the cherry tomatoes in half.

3. In a large bowl, combine the greens, cherry tomatoes , an herbs. Pour the dressing on top and "massage" with your hands

4. Let the greens soak up the dressing. Add more sea sal cayenne pepper, and herbs on top if you wish. Enjoy!

Nutrition:

Calories: 77

Carbohydrates: 11g

Thai Quinoa Salad

Preparation Time: 10 minutes

Cooking Time: 0 minutes

Servings: 1-2

Ingredients :

Ingredients used for dressing:

1 tbsp. Sesame seed

1 tsp. Chopped garlic

1 tsp. Lemon, fresh juice

3 tsp. Apple Cider Vinegar

2 tsp. Tamari, gluten-free.

1/4 cup of tahini (sesame butter)

1 pitted date

1/2 tsp. Salt

1/2 tsp. toasted Sesame oil

Salad Ingredients:

1 cup of quinoa, steamed

1 big handful of arugula

- 1 tomato cut in pieces

- 1/4 of the red onion, diced

Directions:

1. Add the following to a small blender: 1/4 cup + 2 tbsp.

2. Filtered water, the rest of the Ingredients. Blend, man. Steam 1 cup of quinoa in a steamer or a rice pan, then set aside.

3. Combine the quinoa, the arugula, the tomatoes sliced, the red onion diced on a serving plate or bowl, add the Thai dressing

4. and serve with a spoon.

Nutrition:

Calories: 100

Carbohydrates: 12 g

Green Goddess Bowl And Avocado Cumin Dressing

eparation Time: 10 minutes

ooking Time: 0 minutes

ervings: 1-2

gredients :

gredients for the dressing of avocado cumin:

Avocado

tbsp. Cumin Powder

limes, freshly squeezed

cup of filtered water

/4 seconds. sea salt

tbsp. Olive extra virgin olive oil

ayenne pepper dash

Optional: 1/4 tsp. Smoked pepper

hini Lemon Dressing Ingredients

1/4 cup of tahini (sesame butter)

/2 cup of filtered water (more if you want thinner, less thick)

- 1/2 lemon, freshly squeezed

- 1 clove of minced garlic

- 3/4 tsp. Sea salt (Celtic Gray, Himalayan, Redmond Real Salt)

- 1 tbsp. Olive extra virgin olive oil

- black pepper taste

Salad Ingredients:

- 3 cups of kale, chopped

- 1/2 cup of broccoli flowers, chopped

- 1/2 zucchini (make spiral noodles)

- 1/2 cup of kelp noodles, soaked and drained

- 1/3 cup of cherry tomatoes, halved.

- 2 tsp. hemp seeds

Directions:

1. Gently steam the kale and the broccoli (flash the steam for minutes), set aside.

2. Mix the zucchini noodles and kelp noodles and toss with generous portion of the smoked avocado cumin dressing. Ad the cherry tomatoes and stir again.

Place the steamed kale and broccoli and drizzle with the
non tahini dressing. Top the kale and the broccoli with the
odles and tomatoes and sprinkle the whole dish with the
mp seeds.

utrition:

lories: 89

rbohydrates: 11g

t: 1.2g

otein: 4g

Sweet And Savory Salad

Preparation Time: 10 minutes
Cooking Time: 0 minutes
Servings: 1-2

Ingredients :
- 1 big head of butter lettuce

- 1/2 of cucumber, sliced

- 1 pomegranate, seed or 1/3 cup of seed

- 1 avocado, 1 cubed

- 1/4 cup of shelled pistachio, chopped

Ingredients for dressing:

- 1/4 cup of apple cider vinegar

- 1/2 cup of olive oil

- 1 clove of garlic, minced

Directions:
1. Put the butter lettuce in a salad bowl.

. Add the remaining Ingredients and toss with the salad dressing.

Nutrition:

Calories: 68

Carbohydrates: 8g

Fat: 1.2g

Protein: 2g

Beet Salad With Basil Dressing

Preparation Time: 10 minutes
Cooking Time: 0 minutes
Servings: 4

Ingredients :
Ingredients for the dressing

- ¼ cup blackberries

- ¼ cup extra-virgin olive oil

- Juice of 1 lemon

- 2 tablespoons minced fresh basil

- 1 teaspoon poppy seeds

- A pinch of sea salt

- For the salad

- 2 celery stalks, chopped

- 4 cooked beets, peeled and chopped

- 1 cup blackberries

- 4 cups spring mix

Directions:

To make the dressing, mash the blackberries in a bowl. Whisk the oil, lemon juice, basil, poppy seeds, and sea salt.

To make the salad: Add the celery, beets, blackberries, and spring mix to the bowl with the dressing.

Combine and serve.

Nutrition:

Calories: 192

Fat: 15g

Carbohydrates: 15g

Protein: 2g

64

Basic Salad With Olive Oil Dressing

Preparation Time: 10 minutes
Cooking Time: 0 minute
Servings: 4

Ingredients :

• 1 cup coarsely chopped iceberg lettuce

• 1 cup coarsely chopped romaine lettuce

• 1 cup fresh baby spinach

• 1 large tomato, hulled and coarsely chopped

• 1 cup diced cucumber

• 2 tablespoons extra-virgin olive oil

• ¼ teaspoon of sea salt

Directions:

1. In a bowl, combine the spinach and lettuces. Add the tomat and cucumber.

2. Drizzle with oil and sprinkle with sea salt.

3. Mix and serve.

utrition:

lories: 77

t: 4g

rbohydrates: 3g

otein: 1g

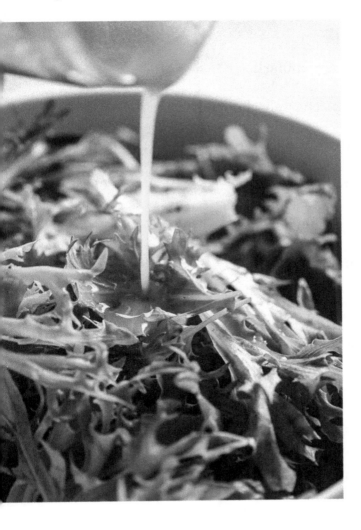

Spinach & Orange Salad With Oi
Drizzle

Preparation Time: 10 minutes
Cooking Time: 0 minute
Servings: 4

Ingredients :

• 4 cups fresh baby spinach

• 1 blood orange, coarsely chopped

• ½ red onion, thinly sliced

• ½ shallot, finely chopped

• 2 tbsp. minced fennel fronds

• Juice of 1 lemon

• 1 tbsp. extra-virgin olive oil

• Pinch sea salt

Directions:

1. In a bowl, toss together the spinach, orange, red onio
shallot, and fennel fronds.

2. Add the lemon juice, oil, and sea salt.

. Mix and serve.

Nutrition:

Calories: 79

Fat: 2g

Carbohydrates: 8g

Protein: 1g

Fruit Salad With Coconut-Lime Dressing

Preparation Time: 5 minutes

Cooking Time: 0 minutes

Servings: 4

Ingredients :

Ingredients for the dressing

- ¼ cup full-fat canned coconut milk

- 1 tbsp. raw honey

- Juice of ½ lime

- Pinch sea salt

- For the salad

- 2 bananas, thinly sliced

- 2 mandarin oranges, segmented

- ½ cup strawberries, thinly sliced

- ½ cup raspberries

- ½ cup blueberries

Directions:

To make the dressing: whisk all the dressing **Ingredients** in bowl.

To make the salad: Add the salad Ingredients in a bowl and mix.

Drizzle with the dressing and serve.

Nutrition:

Calories: 141

Fat: 3g

Carbohydrates: 30g

Protein: 2g

Parsnip, Carrot, And Kale Salad With Dressing

Preparation Time: 10 minutes
Cooking Time: 0 minutes
Servings: 4

Ingredients :
Ingredients for the dressing

• ⅓ cup extra-virgin olive oil

• Juice of 1 lime

• 2 tbsp. minced fresh mint leaves

• 1 tsp. pure maple syrup

• Pinch sea salt

For the salad

• 1 bunch kale, chopped

• ½ parsnip, grated

• ½ carrot, grated

• 2 tbsp. sesame seeds

rections:

To make the dressing, mix all the dressing Ingredients in a wl.

To make the salad, add the kale to the dressing and massage ₂ dressing into the kale for 1 minute.

Add the parsnip, carrot, and sesame seeds.

Combine and serve.

ıtrition:

lories: 214

t: 2g

rbohydrates: 12g

otein: 2g

Tomato Toasts

Preparation Time: 5 minutes
Cooking Time: 5 minutes
Servings: 4

Ingredients :

• 4 slices of sprouted bread toasts

• 2 tomatoes, sliced

• 1 avocado, mashed

• 1 teaspoon olive oil

• 1 pinch of salt

• ¾ teaspoon ground black pepper

Directions:

1. Blend together the olive oil, mashed avocado, salt, and groun
black pepper.

2. When the mixture is homogenous – spread it over th
sprouted bread.

3. Then place the sliced tomatoes over the toasts.

4. Enjoy!

Nutrition:

Calories: 125

Fat: 11.1g

Carbohydrates: 7.0g

Protein: 1.5g

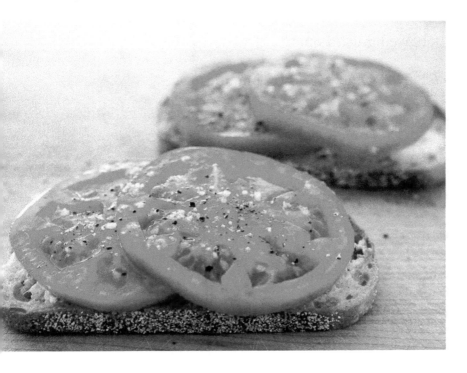

Everyday Salad

Preparation Time: 10 minutes
Cooking Time: 40 minutes
Servings: 6

Ingredients :

• 5 halved mushrooms

• 6 halved Cherry (Plum) Tomatoes

• 6 rinsed Lettuce Leaves

• 10 olives

• ½ chopped cucumber

• Juice from ½ Key Lime

• 1 teaspoon olive oil

• Pure Sea Salt

Directions:

1. Tear rinsed lettuce leaves into medium pieces and put them in a medium salad bowl.

Add mushrooms halves, chopped cucumber, olives and cherry mato halves into the bowl. Mix well. Pour olive and Key Lime ice over salad.

Add pure sea salt to taste. Mix it all till it is well combined.

utrition:

lories: 88

rbohydrates: 11g

t: .5g

otein: .8g

Super-Seedy Salad With Tahini Dressing

Preparation Time: 10 minutes

Cooking Time: 0 minutes

Servings: 1-2

Ingredients :

• 1 slice stale sourdough, torn into chunks

• 50g mixed seeds

• 1 tsp. cumin seeds

• 1 tsp. coriander seeds

• 50g baby kale

• 75g long-stemmed broccoli, blanched for a few minutes the roughly chopped

• ½ red onion, thinly sliced

• 100g cherry tomatoes, halved

• ½ a small bunch flat-leaf parsley, torn

DRESSING

• 100ml natural yogurt

tbsp. tahini

lemon, juiced

rections:

Heat the oven to 200°C/fan 180°C/gas 6. Put the bread into a
od processor and pulse into very rough breadcrumbs. Put into
owl with the mixed seeds and spices, season, and spray well
th oil. Tip onto a non-stick baking tray and roast for 15-20
nutes, stirring and tossing regularly, until deep golden brown.

Whisk together the dressing Ingredients, some seasoning
d a splash of water in a large bowl. Tip the baby kale, broccoli,
1 onion, cherry tomatoes and flat-leaf parsley into the
essing, and mix well. Divide between 2 plates and top with the
spy breadcrumbs and seeds.

utrition:

lories: 78

rbohydrates: 6 g

t: 2g

otein: 1.5g

Vegetable Salad

Preparation Time: 10 minutes

Cooking Time: 0 minutes

Servings: 1-2

Ingredients :

• 4 cups each of raw spinach and romaine lettuce

• 2 cups each of cherry tomatoes, sliced cucumber, chopp(
baby carrots and chopped red, orange and yellow bell pepper

• 1 cup each of chopped broccoli, sliced yellow squash, zucchi
and cauliflower.

Directions:

3. Wash all these vegetables.

4. Mix in a large mixing bowl and top off with a non-fat or lo
fat dressing of your choice.

Nutrition:

Calories: 48

Carbohydrates: 11g

Protein: 3g

Roasted Greek Salad

Preparation Time: 10 minutes

Cooking Time: 0 minutes

Servings: 1-2

Ingredients :

1 Romaine head, torn in bits

1 cucumber sliced

1 pint cherry tomatoes, halved

1 green pepper, thinly sliced

1 onion sliced into rings

1 cup kalamata olives

1 ½ cups feta cheese, crumbled

For dressing combine:

1 cup olive oil

1/4 cup lemon juice

2 tsp. oregano

Salt and pepper

Directions:

1. Lay Ingredients on plate.

2. Drizzle dressing over salad

Nutrition:

Calories: 107

Carbohydrates: 18g

Fat: 1.2 g

Protein: 1g

Alkaline Spring Salad

Preparation Time: 10 minutes

Cooking Time: 0 minutes

Servings: 1-2

Eating seasonal fruits and vegetables is a fabulous way of taking care of yourself and the environment at the same time. This alkaline-electric salad is delicious and nutritious.

Ingredients :

4 cups seasonal approved greens of your choice

1 cup cherry tomatoes

1/4 cup walnuts

1/4 cup approved herbs of your choice

For the dressing:

3-4 key limes

1 tbsp. of homemade raw sesame

Sea salt and cayenne pepper

Directions:

5. First, get the juice of the key limes. In a small bowl, whis together the key lime juice with the homemade raw sesam "tahini" butter. Add sea salt and cayenne pepper, to taste.

6. Cut the cherry tomatoes in half.

7. In a large bowl, combine the greens, cherry tomatoes , an herbs. Pour the dressing on top and "massage" with your hands

8. Let the greens soak up the dressing. Add more sea sal cayenne pepper, and herbs on top if you wish. Enjoy!

Nutrition:

Calories: 77

Carbohydrates: 11g

Tuna Salad

Preparation Time: 10 minutes

Cooking Time: none

Servings: 3

Ingredients :

1 can tuna (6 oz.)

1/3 cup fresh cucumber, chopped

1/3 cup fresh tomato, chopped

1/3 cup avocado, chopped

1/3 cup celery, chopped

2 garlic cloves, minced

4 tsp. olive oil

2 tbsp. lime juice

Pinch of black pepper

Directions:

Prepare the dressing by combining olive oil, lime juice, minced garlic and black pepper.

2. Mix the salad Ingredients in a salad bowl and drizzle with the dressing.

Nutrition:

Carbohydrates: 4.8 g

Protein: 14.3 g

Total sugars: 1.1 g

Calories: 212 g

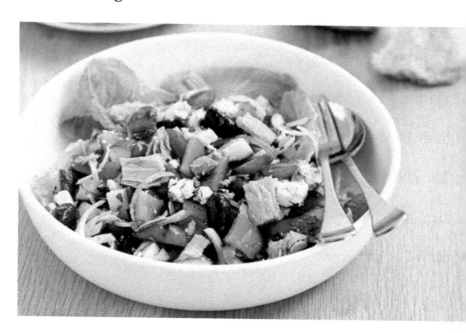

Roasted Portobello Salad

reparation Time: 10 minutes

ooking Time: none

ervings: 4

ngredients :

11/2 lb. Portobello mushrooms, stems trimmed

3 heads Belgian endive, sliced

1 small red onion, sliced

4 oz. blue cheese

8 oz. mixed salad greens

Dressing:

3 tbsp. red wine vinegar

1 tbsp. Dijon mustard

Servings cup olive oil

Salt and pepper to taste

irections:

. Preheat the oven to 450F.

2. Prepare the dressing by whisking together vinegar, mustard salt and pepper. Slowly add olive oil while whisking.

3. Cut the mushrooms and arrange them on a baking sheet stem-side up. Coat the mushrooms with some dressing and bake for 15 minutes.

4. In a salad bowl toss the salad greens with onion, endive and cheese. Sprinkle with the dressing.

5. Add mushrooms to the salad bowl.

Nutrition:

Carbohydrates: 22.3 g

Protein: 14.9 g

Total sugars: 2.1 g

Calories: 501

Shredded Chicken Salad

eparation Time: 5 minutes

ooking Time: 10 minutes

ervings: 6

gredients :

2 chicken breasts, boneless, skinless

1 head iceberg lettuce, cut into strips

2 bell peppers, cut into strips

1 fresh cucumber, quartered, sliced

3 scallions, sliced

2 tbsp. chopped peanuts

1 tbsp. peanut vinaigrette

Salt to taste

1 cup water

irections:

In a skillet simmer one cup of salted water.

2. Add the chicken breasts, cover and cook on low for 5 minute Remove the cover. Then remove the chicken from the skillet ar shred with a fork.

3. In a salad bowl mix the vegetables with the cooled chicke season with salt and sprinkle with peanut vinaigrette ar chopped peanuts.

Nutrition:

Carbohydrates: 9 g

Protein: 11.6 g

Total sugars: 4.2 g

Calories: 117

Cherry Tomato Salad

eparation Time: 10 minutes

oking Time: none

rvings: 6

gredients :

o cherry tomatoes, halved

cup mozzarella balls, halved

cup green olives, sliced

can (6 oz.) black olives, sliced

green onions, chopped

oz. roasted pine nuts

Dressing:

/2 cup olive oil

tbsp. red wine vinegar

tsp. dried oregano

Salt and pepper to taste

rections:

1. In a salad bowl, combine the tomatoes, olives and onions.

2. Prepare the dressing by combining olive oil with red wii vinegar, dried oregano, salt and pepper.

3. Sprinkle with the dressing and add the nuts.

4. Let marinate in the fridge for 15 minutes.

Nutrition:

Carbohydrates: 10.7 g

Protein: 2.4 g

Total sugars: 3.6 g

Ground Turkey Salad

reparation Time: 10 minutes

ooking Time: 35 minutes

ervings: 6

1gredients :

1 lb. lean ground turkey

1/2 inch ginger, minced

2 garlic cloves, minced

1 onion, chopped

1 tbsp. olive oil

1 bag lettuce leaves (for serving)

¼ cup fresh cilantro, chopped

2 tsp. coriander powder

1 tsp. red chili powder

1 tsp. turmeric powder

Salt to taste

4 cups water

Dressing:

- 2 tbsp. fat free yogurt

- 1 tbsp. sour cream, non-fat

- 1 tbsp. low fat mayonnaise

- 1 lemon, juiced

- 1 tsp. red chili flakes

- Salt and pepper to taste

Directions:

1. In a skillet sauté the garlic and ginger in olive oil for 1 minute. Add onion and season with salt. Cook for 10 minutes over medium heat.

2. Add the ground turkey and sauté for 3 more minutes. Add the spices (turmeric, red chili powder and coriander powder).

3. Add 4 cups water and cook for 30 minutes, covered.

4. Prepare the dressing by combining yogurt, sour cream, mayo, lemon juice, chili flakes, salt and pepper.

5. To serve arrange the salad leaves on serving plates and place the cooked ground turkey on them. Top with dressing.

Nutrition:

Carbohydrates: 9.1 g

Protein: 17.8 g

Total sugars: 2.5 g

Calories: 176

Asian Cucumber Salad

Preparation Time: 10 minutes

Cooking Time: none

Servings: 6

Ingredients :

- 1 lb. cucumbers, sliced

- 2 scallions, sliced

- 2 tbsp. sliced pickled ginger, chopped

- ¼ cup cilantro

- 1/2 red jalapeño, chopped

- 3 tbsp. rice wine vinegar

- 1 tbsp. sesame oil

- 1 tbsp. sesame seeds

Directions:

1. In a salad bowl combine all Ingredients and toss together.

Nutrition:

Carbohydrates: 5.7 g

otein: 1 g

tal sugars: 3.1 g

lories: 52

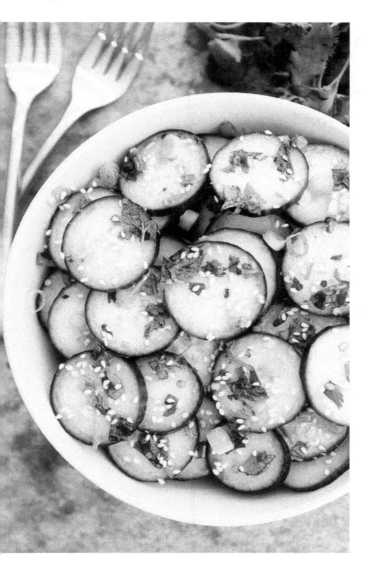

Cauliflower Tofu Salad

Preparation Time: 10 minutes

Cooking Time: 15 minutes

Servings: 4

Ingredients :

• 2 cups cauliflower florets, blended

• 1 fresh cucumber, diced

• 1/2 cup green olives, diced

• 1/3 cup red onion, diced

• 2 tbsp. toasted pine nuts

• 2 tbsp. raisins

• 1/3 cup feta, crumbled

• 1/2 cup pomegranate seeds

• 2 lemons (juiced, zest grated)

• 8 oz. tofu

• 2 tsp. oregano

• 2 garlic cloves, minced

1/2 tsp. red chili flakes

3 tbsp. olive oil

Salt and pepper to taste

Directions:

. Season the processed cauliflower with salt and transfer to a strainer to drain.

. Prepare the marinade for tofu by combining 2 tbsp. lemon juice, 1.5 tbsp. olive oil, minced garlic, chili flakes, oregano, salt and pepper. Coat tofu in the marinade and set aside.

. Preheat the oven to 450F.

. Bake tofu on a baking sheet for 12 minutes.

. In a salad bowl mix the remaining marinade with onions, cucumber, cauliflower, olives and raisins. Add in the remaining olive oil and grated lemon zest.

. Top with tofu, pine nuts, and feta and pomegranate seeds.

Nutrition:

Carbohydrates: 34.1 g

Protein: 11.1 g

Total sugars: 11.5 g

Calories: 328

Scallop Caesar Salad

Preparation Time: 5 minutes

Cooking Time: 2 minutes

Servings: 2

Ingredients :

• 8 sea scallops

• 4 cups romaine lettuce

• 2 tsp. olive oil

• 3 tbsp. Caesar Salad Dressing

• 1 tsp. lemon juice

• Salt and pepper to taste

Directions:

1. In a frying pan heat olive oil and cook the scallops in one layer no longer than 2 minutes per both sides. Season with salt and pepper to taste.

2. Arrange lettuce on plates and place scallops on top.

3. Pour over the Caesar dressing and lemon juice.

Nutrition:

Carbohydrates: 14 g

Protein: 30.7 g

Total sugars: 2.2 g

Calories: 340 g

Chicken Avocado Salad

Preparation Time: 30 minutes

Cooking Time: 15 minutes

Servings: 4

Ingredients :

• 1 lb. chicken breast, cooked, shredded

• 1 avocado, pitted, peeled, sliced

• 2 tomatoes, diced

• 1 cucumber, peeled, sliced

• 1 head lettuce, chopped

• 3 tbsp. olive oil

• 2 tbsp. lime juice

• 1 tbsp. cilantro, chopped

• Salt and pepper to taste

Directions:

1. In a bowl whisk together oil, lime juice, cilantro, salt, and pinch of pepper.

Combine lettuce, tomatoes, cucumber in a salad bowl and ss with half of the dressing.

Toss chicken with the remaining dressing and combine with getable mixture.

Top with avocado.

itrition:

rbohydrates: 10 g

otein: 38 g

tal sugars: 11.5 g

lories: 380

California Wraps

Preparation Time: 5 minutes

Cooking Time: 15 minutes

Servings: 4

Ingredients :

• 4 slices turkey breast, cooked

• 4 slices ham, cooked

• 4 lettuce leaves

• 4 slices tomato

• 4 slices avocado

• 1 tsp. lime juice

• A handful watercress leaves

• 4 tbsp. Ranch dressing, sugar free

Directions:

1. Top a lettuce leaf with turkey slice, ham slice and tomato.

2. In a bowl combine avocado and lime juice and place on top tomatoes. Top with water cress and dressing.

. Repeat with the remaining Ingredients for

. Topping each lettuce leaf with a turkey slice, ham slice, mato and dressing.

utrition:

arbohydrates: 4 g

rotein: 9 g

otal sugars: 0.5 g

alories: 140

Chicken Salad In Cucumber Cups

Preparation Time: 5 minutes

Cooking Time: 15 minutes

Servings: 4

Ingredients :

• 1/2 chicken breast, skinless, boiled and shredded

• 2 long cucumbers, cut into 8 thick rounds each, scooped ou
(won't use in a).

• 1 tsp. ginger, minced

• 1 tsp. lime zest, grated

• 4 tsp. olive oil

• 1 tsp. sesame oil

• 1 tsp. lime juice

• Salt and pepper to taste

Directions:

1. In a bowl combine lime zest, juice, olive and sesame oils
ginger, and season with salt.

Toss the chicken with the dressing and fill the cucumber cups
with the salad.

Nutrition:

Carbohydrates: 4 g

Protein: 12 g

Total sugars: 0.5 g

Calories: 116 g

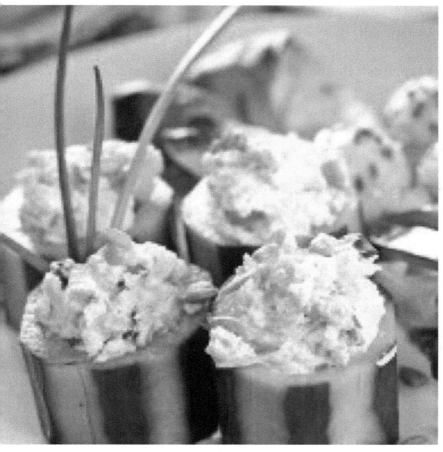

Sunflower Seeds And Arugula Garden Salad

Preparation Time: 5 minutes

Cooking Time: 10 minutes

Servings: 6

Ingredients :

• ¼ tsp. black pepper

• ¼ tsp. salt

• 1 tsp. fresh thyme, chopped

• 2 tbsp. sunflower seeds, toasted

• 2 cups red grapes, halved

• 7 cups baby arugula, loosely packed

• 1 tbsp. coconut oil

• 2 tsp. honey

• 3 tbsp. red wine vinegar

• 1/2 tsp. stone-ground mustard

rections:

In a small bowl, whisk together mustard, honey and vinegar. wly pour oil as you whisk.

In a large salad bowl, mix thyme, seeds, grapes and arugula.

Drizzle with dressing and serve.

utrition:

lories: 86 7g

otein: 1.6g

rbs: 13.1g

t: 3.1g.

Supreme Caesar Salad

Preparation Time: 5 minutes
Cooking Time: 10 minutes
Servings: 4

Ingredients :

• ¼ cup olive oil

• ¾ cup mayonnaise

• 1 head romaine lettuce, torn into bite sized pieces

• 1 tbsp. lemon juice

• 1 tsp. Dijon mustard

• 1 tsp. Worcestershire sauce

• 3 cloves garlic, peeled and minced

• 3 cloves garlic, peeled and quartered

• 4 cups day old bread, cubed

• 5 anchovy filets, minced

• 6 tbsp. grated parmesan cheese, divided

• Ground black pepper to taste

• Salt to taste

Directions:

In a small bowl, whisk well lemon juice, mustard, Worcestershire sauce, 2 tbsp. parmesan cheese, anchovies, mayonnaise, and minced garlic. Season with pepper and salt to taste. Set aside in the ref.

. On medium fire, place a large nonstick saucepan and heat oil.

. Sauté quartered garlic until browned around a minute or two. Remove and discard.

. Add bread cubes in same pan, sauté until lightly browned. Season with pepper and salt. Transfer to a plate.

. In large bowl, place lettuce and pour in dressing. Toss well to coat. Top with remaining parmesan cheese.

. Garnish with bread cubes, serve, and enjoy.

Nutrition:

Calories: 443.3g

Fat: 32.1g

Protein: 11.6g

Carbs: 27g

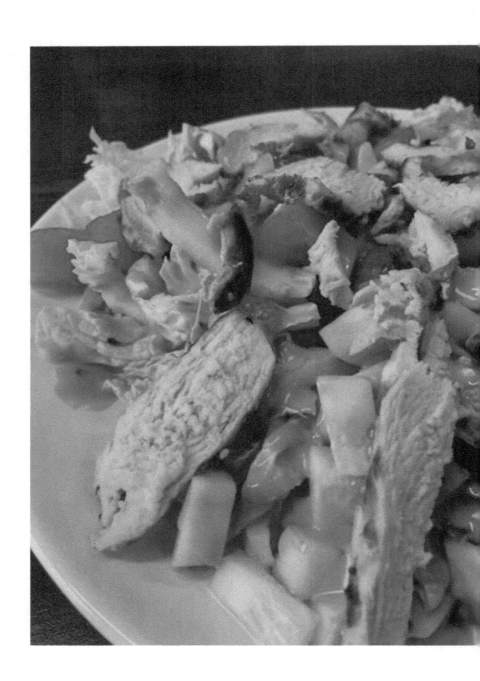